Fuelling the Original AI: Training the Mind, Powering the Body

"Strengthen your mind. Power your body. Command your life."

By Thomas Lashan

Table of Contents

A Note Before We Begin 3

Your Mind Is a Search Engine — Use It Consciously 10

Understanding the Thousands of Thoughts That Shape You Daily 15

Check In, Reset, and Keep Moving 20

Choice Builds AI Efficiency 23

Clutter, The Silent Weight on Your Mind and AI 26

5-Minute Digital Reset Routine 32

A Simple New Rule to Power Your AI 36

Universal Energies — The Invisible Flow That Shapes Us 39

Exercise — Demanding on the Body, Powerful for the Mind 43

The Box Story — Your Inner Sanctuary 51

The Power of Cold Showers: Building Awareness, Resilience, and a Sharper Mind 54

The Invisible Trap of Old Wives' Tales: How Belief Becomes Biology 57

Training Hurdles, Niggles, and The Power of Conscious Control 63

The Body's Goal — And It's Not What You Think 67

Fuel for the Original AI: How Nutrition Drives Mind and Body Efficiency 74

The First Rule of Change: Define the Outcome and Make It Matter 78

Evening Rituals for Reset & Recovery 83

The Power of a Grateful Pause 87

Take the Helm — You Are the CEO of You 91

Periodisation: Training with Purpose and Timing 95

Weight Training Structure, and Nutrition 103

"The mind finds peace not by silencing the world, but by learning to hear itself above the noise." Thomas Lashan

A Note Before We Begin

If you've read Mind: The Original AI (Book One), then you're already aware, awareness is the first step to transformation. But now comes the true challenge: implementation. The moment you decide to take conscious control of your life, it can feel like the world starts to push back. It's not that life is working against you, it's that you're seeing everything through a new lens. You've shifted your perspective, and naturally, everything looks and feels different.

That's because transformation requires movement, and movement stirs resistance, not as punishment, but as preparation.

Imagine you've decided to go on a road trip, short or long, it doesn't matter. You don't just jump in the car and go. You pack, plan, anticipate what might come up. You're not hoping for a flat tyre, bad weather, or delays, but you prepare just in case. And when those challenges do come, you handle them because the destination matters, and the journey is part of it.

Life works the same way. When you commit to a new mindset, a new path, or a new version of yourself, life doesn't test you to stop you, it tests you to shape you. The discomfort you feel is the shedding of the old, the expansion of your capacity, the alignment with who you're becoming.

Let's look at another example: elite athletes. Their goals are clear. Their vision is specific. But the moment they commit, they don't avoid difficulty, they expect it. Every early morning, every injury, every doubt is part of the shaping process. When they finally reach peak performance, it's not in spite of the challenges, it's because of them.

So as you begin this next part of your journey, remember: resistance is not your enemy, it's your training partner. The challenges are not detours, they're the path. And everything that shows up, especially the hard parts, is preparing you for what you asked for.

Book Two is your next step, not just to understand, but to embody. You've unlocked awareness. Now let's build the mindset that can hold the vision.

Make It Easy

This book is designed to be an easy, uncomplicated read, and that's deliberate.

Life already throws enough complexity our way. Between endless decisions, opinions, information, and noise, clarity is rare. So the message within these pages has been kept simple, clear, and open-ended. Why?

Because this isn't a book to box you in. It isn't here to tell you what to believe or how to live. It's here to offer ideas, insights, and practices you can weave into your own story, in your own way.

Let it fuel your curiosity.

Let it spark your creativity.

Take what makes sense to you, and leave what doesn't.

The goal is for these ideas to become tools you shape, not rules you follow.

The Mind's Untapped Power

We've Known It for Centuries… But Rarely Acted on It

For thousands of years, philosophers, mystics and healers have spoken about the mind's influence over the body and the world around it. Ancient Ayurvedic medicine, Traditional Chinese Medicine, Stoic philosophy, Indigenous wisdom, they all carried versions of the same message:

Your thoughts shape your body, your energy, your health, and your outcomes.

Yet in the modern world, we've become disconnected from this truth. We've outsourced our health to specialists, our decision-making to devices, and our inner world to distractions.

While technology and medicine have advanced rapidly, **our ability to master our own mind has stagnated.**

It's not because the mind has become weaker, it's because we've stopped training it.

Modern Science Now Proves What Ancient Wisdom Knew

Today, cutting-edge neuroscience is catching up with what those ancient traditions claimed:

Neuroplasticity:

Studies at Harvard, MIT and Stanford show that the brain physically rewires itself in response to new behaviours, thoughts and experiences. You are not fixed. You can literally reshape your neural connections and emotional patterns at any age.

The Placebo Effect:

It's no coincidence that sugar pills in clinical trials often produce real, measurable changes in health outcomes. The placebo effect is **the subconscious mind's belief in healing triggering physiological improvements** — without any active ingredients. The mind made the body better.

Meditation and Breath work Research:

fMRI studies reveal that even 10 minutes of daily meditation shrinks the brain's fear centre (the amygdala) while increasing the size of the prefrontal cortex — the part responsible for decision-making, focus and calm control.

Breath work has been shown to regulate heart rate variability, lower blood pressure, and activate the parasympathetic nervous system for healing.

Dr. Bruce Lipton's Work (The Biology of Belief):

His research found that the environment surrounding our cells — which includes our thoughts, beliefs, and emotions — controls gene expression.

Meaning: your mindset can literally turn health-promoting or health-damaging genes on or off.

Picture It Like a Pie

To make sense of this, imagine your mind like a pie chart:

- **5% Conscious Mind:**

The voice reading this now. It sets goals, makes plans, and acts on logic, but it's limited in capacity and influence.

- **95% Subconscious Mind:**

This is the control room. It runs your habits, reactions, beliefs, fears, identity, and automatic behaviours. It even regulates your heartbeat and digestion without you thinking about it.

Most people spend their entire lives being run by programs they didn't consciously choose.

And here's the tragedy:

This 95% can be reprogrammed, but most us never try.

A Real-World Story to Prove the Point

Remember Dr. Ellen Langer's famous **Counterclockwise Study** in the 1980s?

A group of elderly men was placed in a setting made to feel like it was 1959. They dressed in 50s clothing, surrounded by magazines and music of the time, and spoke as if it were decades earlier.

The result after one week?

- Improved posture
- Sharper memory
- Greater flexibility and joint function
- Enhanced eyesight
- Measurably younger appearance according to before-and-after photos judged by independent observers.

Why?

Because their subconscious mind believed they were younger, stronger, and freer, so their body followed the instructions.

This is your untapped power. And it's available every day.

Why This Book Exists

This book exists to give you the simple, practical tools to access that 95% of yourself, your personal AI.

It won't require you to meditate in a cave or live in a lab. It's about using small, intentional daily practices, in your breathing, movement, eating, thinking and technology habits, to train your

mind to work with you, not against you.

Each section of this book isn't just advice.

It's a way to rewrite the code your subconscious mind runs on.

A Thought for You as You Begin

"You don't rise to the level of your goals, you fall to the level of your systems."

— James Clear, *Atomic Habits*

Your mind is a system.

Your body is a system.

Your habits are a system.

This book is about upgrading those systems so they finally align with the life you say you want.

Your Mind Is a Search Engine — Use It Consciously

For years, we've relied on search engines like Google to find answers. At the click of a button, we type in a question and it delivers a list of results from everywhere across the internet. It revolutionised how we access knowledge.

Now, AI takes this even further — we no longer just search; we ask, and it thinks for us. It interprets, sorts, prioritize, and delivers.

But what most people forget is that we've always had our own powerful search engine built- in: **the conscious mind.**

How Your Internal Search Engine Works

Your mind is constantly processing — somewhere between **60,000 to 70,000 thoughts per day** according to studies from the National Science Foundation. Most of these are subconscious background noise unless you choose to consciously focus.

Here's where the analogy is powerful:

- **When you ask yourself a question, your mind immediately starts searching for an answer.**

This can be memory-based, feeling-based, or even creative problem-solving.

- Just like a search engine, **the quality of your question**

determines the quality of the answer you get.

Ask poor, fear-based questions like *"Why does this always happen to me?"* and your mind will search for evidence to justify that.

Ask constructive, growth-based questions like *"What can I learn here to grow stronger?"* — and your mind searches for helpful, empowering data.

Your Conscious Mind: The AI Operator

Now, think of your conscious mind like the operator of both your external search engines (Google, AI tools) **and your internal subconscious library.**

It decides what to type in.

It decides which results to click.

It chooses whether to dwell on something negative or redirect to a constructive alternative.

Why This Matters to Your AI Training

The smoother your conscious mind can direct your internal 'search engine,' the clearer and calmer your decision-making becomes.

Your mind, like AI, works best when:

- It knows what to look for (clear intentions)
- It can ignore irrelevant results (mental discipline)

- It's regularly cleaned of outdated or toxic data (old limiting beliefs)

Just like updating your phone or clearing browser history for faster performance — you need to routinely update, declutter and consciously direct your internal processing.

Food for Thought

If AI can scour the world's information for you, and your mind can access decades of personal experience, then the only limit is your clarity in asking the right question.

Whether you're searching for answers online or within yourself, the one skill you'll always need is **conscious, intentional questioning.**

That's the key to becoming your own AI architect.

Reflection Exercise: Train Your Inner Search Engine

We've just explored how your mind operates like a search engine, or better yet, like your personal AI system. The strength of your thinking, mood, and decision-making depends heavily on the **quality of the questions you habitually ask yourself.**

So now, let's make this real for you.

Step 1: Audit the Questions You Ask Daily

Take a moment and honestly list some of the automatic or common thoughts you catch yourself repeating.

- Why does this always happen to me?

- I wonder what people think of me.

- Why can't I ever catch a break?

- How can I get ahead this week?

- What am I grateful for today?

- How can I improve by 1% today?

Notice how some of these feel **heavy and limiting**, while others feel **empowering and forward-moving**.

Step 2: Categorise Them

Now, sort your questions into these three groups:

- **Disempowering Questions** (the ones that reinforce limitation or victim mindset)

- **Neutral Questions** (functional, everyday survival stuff)

- **Empowering Questions** (the ones that help you grow, learn, or improve)

This shows you what your mind is 'searching' for all day.

Step 3: Upgrade Your Questions

Replace disempowering or wasteful questions with constructive alternatives. For example:

❌ *Why am I so tired?*

✅ *What can I do today to boost my energy naturally?*

❌ *Why can't I ever win?*

✅ *What can I learn from this to improve my chances next time?*

This is AI training in action.

The better your conscious mind becomes at asking quality questions, the more precise and productive your internal AI becomes.

Takeaway Thought

"The questions you ask yourself set the direction of your mind's search engine. Train it wisely, and it will deliver outcomes beyond what you believed possible."

Understanding the Thousands of Thoughts That Shape You Daily

Modern neuroscience confirms that the average human mind generates **between 6,000 to 70,000 thoughts per day**. The variation depends on how researchers measure a "thought," but studies like those conducted at **Queen's University in Canada (2020)** have found a conservative, trackable number around **6,200 distinct thought transitions a day**.

Now — imagine for a moment that every one of those thoughts is an instruction your subconscious AI is processing, tagging, and filing away. The vast majority go unnoticed, but they shape your mood, choices, energy, and ultimately, your reality.

To sharpen your AI, you must become aware of the types of thoughts you're having and learn to filter or redirect them. I like to break these down into **four simple groups:**

Necessary Thoughts

These are the functional, life-operating thoughts. They help you:

- Wake up on time
- Prepare breakfast
- Remember your schedule
- Navigate conversations
- Pay bills

- They keep your life moving and are essential for daily survival. You don't need to overly interfere with these, they're helpful, practical, and largely automatic.

Waste Thoughts

This is where most people burn precious energy and mental clarity. Waste thoughts fall into two main camps:

a) **Dwelling on the Past:**

Reliving past mistakes, arguments, regrets, or even old victories to self-soothe or punish. Unless you're consciously extracting a lesson to use now, it's dead weight. This is mental rubbish you carry, and the AI keeps running these programs unless you instruct it to stop.

b) **Worrying About the Future:**

The *what ifs* that have no foundation in present action:

- *What if that meeting goes badly?*
- *What if I get sick?*
- *What if they don't like me?*

While *planning* for a future event is productive, **excessive speculation without action is wasted processing power**. It clouds judgment, feeds anxiety, and creates imaginary outcomes that often never happen.

Studies from the National Science Foundation (2005) found that **around 80% of our daily thoughts are negative, and 95% are**

repetitive. Most of this comes from waste thought loops about past and future situations we can't control.

Positive, Growth-Based Thoughts

These are conscious, intentional thoughts that serve your development:

- *I'm getting stronger each day.*
- *This challenge is teaching me something valuable.*
- *I have the power to reshape my future.*
- *What is one thing I can do better today?*

Positive thoughts fuel your AI to operate from a space of expansion, clarity, and courage. They elevate your frequency, literally changing your biochemistry through dopamine, serotonin, and oxytocin release.

These thoughts build resilience, creative problem-solving, and mental toughness. The more you repeat them, the more your subconscious accepts them as default.

Negative, Limiting Thoughts

These thoughts are silent assassins. Left unchecked, they wear down your self-belief and block you from growth:

- *I'll never be able to do this.*

- *I'm not good enough.*

- *Why bother? Nothing changes anyway.*

- *They probably don't like me.*

Even fleeting, these thoughts leave imprints. Every repetition is like coding faulty software into your AI. What's worse, **the subconscious cannot tell the difference between a joke, sarcasm, or deliberate self-talk** — it absorbs all input as fact.

Dr. Bruce Lipton, cellular biologist and author of *The Biology of Belief*, has shown how negative thought patterns alter genetic expression and impact physical health, immune response, and neural wiring.

Exercise: Thought Audit, 24-Hour Mind Cleanse

Purpose:

To gain awareness of your thought patterns, identify mental clutter, and begin reshaping your internal AI for clarity, focus, and personal power.

Instructions:

For the next **24 hours**, become an observer of your own mind. Every time you catch yourself thinking something, pause and mentally sort it into one of the four categories:

- 🔘 **Necessary Thought**

(Keeps you functioning, practical, no problem.)

- ⬤ **Waste Thought**

(Dwelling on past regrets, pointless future worries, or things outside your control.)

- ◐ **Positive, Growth-Based Thought**

(Uplifting, focused on progress, solutions, gratitude, or opportunity.)

- ⬤ **Negative, Limiting Thought**

(Self-doubt, criticism, defeatist thinking, or harmful predictions.)

Quick Tip:

If you struggle to catch yourself in real-time, take **5 minutes every evening** to reflect on your day and jot down a few examples in each category.

Reflection Questions (End of Day)

- What category dominated your thinking today?
- Which waste thoughts kept looping in your mind?
- How did your positive thoughts make you feel in your body?
- What one limiting thought do you want to catch and redirect tomorrow?

Next-Level Challenge:

If you're game, make it your mission to **turn every waste or negative**

thought into a positive reframe. For example:

Instead of:

"This is too hard."

Say:

"This challenge will grow me."

And notice what happens to your energy.

"A well-managed mind is a life well-designed."

Check In, Reset, and Keep Moving

Before we dive into this next chapter of your growth, take a breath. Check in with yourself. How's the journey so far? Have you noticed yourself pausing before reacting? Noticing old patterns as they surface? Catching those internal conversations that no longer serve you?

If you have, even once, you're on track. And if it feels slow, messy, or inconsistent, you're still on track. That's how real, lasting change works. It's never instant, but always worthwhile.

Practice is the bridge between where you are and where you want to be

Along that bridge, setbacks aren't detours, they're confirmations. Every time you stumble or slip into an old habit, it's life showing you contrast. It's evidence that you no longer want that version of yourself, and a reminder to return to the path.

That's why **Mind: The Original AI** was written intentionally short. Not because your growth is small, but because simplicity is powerful. You're meant to revisit it often, flick it open to a page, absorb what you need in that moment, and carry on a little stronger than before.

Let's ground this idea with something you'll recognise.

Imagine deciding to start walking or running for your well-being. You don't head out for one jog and think, *"Great, I'm healthy for life."* The benefits aren't in the single act, but in the rhythm of it. Every walk or run makes the next one easier. The muscles strengthen. The mind gets clearer. The results are compound.

And so it is with your inner world. The more you challenge old thoughts, the more you choose calm over chaos, courage over fear, truth over excuses, the stronger your mind, your original AI, becomes.

And be mindful, the challenges you face aren't random. You asked for change. Life answered with opportunities dressed up as obstacles. Every setback isn't there to punish you. It's there to prepare you.

Here is an analogy

You plan, shop for, and carefully prepare a beautiful, nourishing meal. The colours are perfect, the aroma irresistible, the nutrients exactly what your body needs. But then… you don't eat it. You leave it on the plate.

That's what it's like to ask for a better life, to gather knowledge, read books, attend workshops, and then refuse to practice any of it. Don't be the person who makes the meal but starves anyway.

Your life will change when your actions catch up to your intentions.

And to leave you with a thought as we move forward:

"Your mind is the original technology. Learn to program it well, and you'll no longer chase peace, you'll generate it."

The Power of Choice: Training Your AI Mind to Lead

When it comes to choosing your training and nutrition path, the most important rule is this:

It must come from you. Why?

Because when you do the work to research, test, and discover what aligns with your body, your mind, and your life, that's not just success, that's power. It's agency. It's your Original AI learning, adapting, and strengthening through experience.

Think of it like going to the gym: no one else can lift the weights for you. Not your friends, not your family. **This is your gift to yourself.**

And few things in life are more satisfying than knowing *you earned it, you chose it, you built it.*

Choice Builds AI Efficiency

Every time you make a conscious choice for your body, your training, your nutrition, or your mindset, you're programming your AI.

You're teaching it how to respond in the future.

You're building an efficient system that makes aligned, confident decisions faster, clearer, and without hesitation.

This is how leaders are made. Not by avoiding choice, but by leaning into it.

In My Coaching Days…

When I trained clients, I never dictated every move. Sure, I guided them, but I always gave them choices. Why?

Because **choice is power**.

And it's through making choices, even small ones, that we claim ownership of our journey.

I wasn't there to count their reps for glory.

I was there to help them see that every decision was a chance to get stronger, inside and out.

In This Book…

I'll offer suggestions, frameworks, and proven ideas. But ultimately, **you must choose.**

And when you do, when you own that decision… watch how your internal AI sharpens, accelerates, and begins to lead your life for you.

Because choice isn't just action, it's reprogramming.

And every smart decision is another upgrade.

Breathing: The Power and the Support

If there's one practice to master, it's your **breathing,** because it's the bridge between your conscious mind and your Original AI.

Breathing through the nose is your power.

It calms the nervous system, sharpens focus, regulates the heart rate, and keeps you connected to yourself in the present moment. Throughout your day, nose breathing is how you anchor your mind, steady your emotions, and stay in tune with your AI's guidance.

But during **training**, there's a different rule.

When intensity rises and the demand on your system increases, **mouth breathing becomes the support system**. It helps you move more oxygen quickly, clear carbon dioxide faster, and keep your body performing under load.

The key is to use both with intention:

- **Nose breathing** for power, when you need calm, control, clarity.

- **Mouth breathing** for support, when you need to dig deep, recover, and push through effort.

When you become aware of this, you start to train your breathing the same way you train your muscles or your mindset. It becomes a tool, not just a function.

Master this, and you'll notice everything else improves:

- Your mental clarity

- Your decision-making under pressure

- Your recovery

- And most importantly, your connection to your AI, the part of you that's always working for your highest good.

Own your breath, and you own the moment.

Clutter, The Silent Weight on Your Mind and AI

We often underestimate how much our **physical environment mirrors our internal state**. Clutter isn't just about mess. It's about **energy congestion**. Every time you walk past the overstuffed garage, the kitchen bench piled with unopened mail, or the spare room you keep meaning to tidy, your subconscious registers it as an unresolved task. Whether you're aware of it or not, that mental bookmark adds a small weight to your mind, and over time, those small weights compound.

Studies in neuroscience have shown that visual clutter competes for your attention, reduces your working memory, and can increase cortisol levels, the stress hormone, making you feel more anxious and less focused. A 2011 study by the Princeton Neuroscience Institute found that people surrounded by physical clutter were **less productive, more easily distracted, and more likely to procrastinate.**

But it's not just about productivity, it's about **clarity**. When our environment feels chaotic, so does our mind. When our external world is overwhelmed, our **inner AI** is forced to allocate bandwidth to constantly process and dismiss those unresolved 'to-do's'.

Mindful Clutter Check

- Is there a drawer, cupboard, or room you avoid?
- Are you 'used to' the mess but feel a little drained when you

notice it?

- Do you often say "I need to sort that out" — but don't?

If yes, that's not just junk. That's unspent mental energy, weighing down your processing power.

Why Clearing Clutter Is More Than Cleaning

When you consciously choose to clear, organise, or even throw out what no longer serves you, you send a clear message to your mind:

"I'm in control of my space, my time, and my life."

It instantly lightens your subconscious load, creating more space for clarity, focus, and confidence. It's not about having a picture-perfect home, it's about removing the subconscious obstacles that quietly drain your motivation and awareness.

Quick Exercise:

Pick **one small area** today, a drawer, your car, a bench top, and clear it. Not because you have to, but to experience how much lighter your mind feels when you remove one small weight from your subconscious.

"Your environment whispers to your mind all day long. Make sure it's saying something empowering."

Digital Clutter — The Invisible Mental Drain

In a world where our lives are increasingly played out through screens, **digital clutter has become one of the biggest invisible stressors we**

carry. And the problem is, it's always with us, in our pockets, on our desks, and even on our wrists.

Unread emails, hundreds of unsorted photos, dozens of browser tabs left open, notification pings, and half-finished to-do lists in five different apps, all these micro-clutters quietly pile up in your subconscious.

Just like physical mess, digital clutter signals **unfinished business** to your brain, and your inner AI quietly logs those unresolved loops. Whether you're consciously aware of it or not, it erodes clarity, adds low-level anxiety, and eats away at your mental efficiency.

Take a Moment in the Noise

We're living in the most information-saturated era in history, especially when it comes to health, diet, and training. Open your phone and within seconds you're hit with advice from all directions: "Cut carbs," "Train faster," "Only eat clean," "Supplements are essential," and so on. And while some of this may come from well-meaning people, much of it is unfiltered, unproven, or based on personal experience dressed up as universal truth.

The problem isn't just the volume, it's the confusion it creates. One post leads to another opinion, which then spawns more content layered with further interpretation. The truth, somewhere in the middle, becomes blurry. This isn't a dig at anyone, we've all shared what worked for us. But here's the key insight: what works for one person, at one stage of life, doesn't automatically work for everyone else.

Take diet, for example. It's easy for a 20-something with a high metabolism and active lifestyle to say "cut carbs" or "just eat clean." But for someone in their 40s, 50s or 60s, navigating hormone shifts, stress, slower recovery, and real metabolic challenges, that advice might not just be unhelpful, it might be harmful.

So here's the shift:

Rather than letting yourself be pulled and prodded by every new piece of advice, come back to your own internal guidance system, your original AI. Your body is speaking. Your energy, your mood, your sleep, your recovery, these are all feedback loops. By quieting the digital noise, tuning in, and layering in science-based understanding, you begin to reclaim the most accurate health compass there is: you.

We're not saying ignore everything, but question what you consume, digitally and physically. Awareness + curiosity + personal tracking = clarity.

That's how we move from confusion to confidence. That's how we build a sustainable, powerful way forward.

What Research Tells Us

A study from the University of California Irvine found that office workers took **an average of 23 minutes to regain focus** after a digital interruption. Now imagine those interruptions happening dozens of times a day.

Additionally, researchers at Princeton Neuroscience Institute discovered that **clutter — physical or digital — competes for your attention and reduces your brain's ability to focus and process information.**

This means every unread notification, crowded desktop, and cluttered inbox isn't harmless

— it's actively slowing down your ability to think clearly, make decisions, and stay aligned with your goals.

Decluttering Your Digital Space: A Mindful Ritual

- **Tidy Your Phone Home Screen:** Remove unused apps, sort remaining ones into folders, and leave only what adds value or peace.

- **Clean Out Your Inbox:** Unsubscribe from junk mail, delete old promotions, and create folders for key categories.

- **Close All Tabs:** End each workday by closing unnecessary browser tabs. It's like clearing your desk before you leave.

- **Turn Off Notifications:** Decide which apps *really* need to interrupt your focus. Hint: it's probably a lot less than you think.

- **Digital Sabbath:** Take a few hours a week, even one afternoon, where your phone stays out of sight.

Why This Matters to Your AI Development

When you remove digital clutter, you free up **mental bandwidth**. More space for creativity. More clarity for decision-making. More present moments where your AI can process quality data instead of digital noise.

This act of conscious control over your digital world tells your inner AI,

"I decide what gets my attention."

That one belief, when exercised daily, will sharpen your awareness, improve emotional resilience, and strengthen the decision-making muscle that shapes your future.

"Attention is your most valuable currency. Spend it wisely, and invest it where it pays you back in peace, clarity, and growth."

5-Minute Digital Reset Routine

A simple, mindful exercise you can do once a day, or even just a few times a week, to reclaim your focus and clean your mental space.

Step 1: Home Screen Audit (1 minute)

- Look at your phone home screen.
- **Remove one app you haven't used in a month.**

If you hesitate, you probably don't need it.

Step 2: Email & Notifications Sweep (1 minute)

- Open your inbox, delete or archive **10 emails** you'll never action.
- Unsubscribe from one useless newsletter.
- Turn off notifications for any app that isn't essential to your work, health, or family.

Step 3: Close Tabs & Apps (1 minute)

- On your computer and phone, **close every tab or app you don't need open right now.**
- Ask yourself, *"Is this helping or distracting me?"*

If it's not helping — close it.

Step 4: Digital Gratitude (1 minute)

- Pick one digital tool, app, or person you connect with online that's added value to your life this week.
- Pause and consciously feel gratitude for it.
- This rewires your mind to recognize and prioritise positive digital habits.

Step 5: Set One Digital Boundary (1 minute)

- Choose **one boundary for today**:
  - No phone at meals.
  - No social media before bed.
  - 20 minutes of screen-free time after lunch.
- Mentally commit to it.

This tells your AI you're in charge.

Why This Works

By regularly reclaiming control over your digital world, you send a clear message to your subconscious:

"I choose what enters my space, what holds my attention, and what energy I carry."

This small, consistent practice sharpens awareness, boosts decision-making clarity, and lifts your daily mental energy, creating compounding benefits for your AI development and life momentum.

The Power of Sleep in Sharpening Your AI

One of the most overlooked tools in upgrading your inner operating system — your AI — is sleep. It's not just rest for the body; it's critical maintenance for the mind. The simple truth is this: when you compromise on sleep, you compromise on clarity, focus, emotional balance, and your ability to make sound decisions. And while one bad night might not ruin you, poor sleep habits over time can distort your thought processes and decision-making abilities, setting you back days, even weeks in your efforts to strengthen your AI.

Here's why:

During quality sleep, particularly in the deep (slow-wave) and REM phases, the brain performs a series of essential processes:

- **Information consolidation:** It takes what you've learned, felt, and experienced during the day and organises it. New skills are encoded, emotional experiences are processed, and subconscious programs are subtly updated.

- **Emotional regulation:** The amygdala, the brain's emotional control centre, becomes hyperactive with sleep deprivation. This means you're more likely to react emotionally, less likely to pause and make conscious, considered decisions.

- **Detox and repair:** Your brain clears out metabolic waste through the glymphatic system during sleep. Without enough rest, these waste products accumulate — literally clouding your mind and slowing cognitive performance.

Studies have shown:

- People who get less than six hours of sleep for just one week experience a drop in attention, memory recall, and problem-solving ability equivalent to ageing the brain by up to five years.

- Decision-making accuracy declines by up to **50%** after 18–24 hours of sleep deprivation, according to research from the **Cognitive Neuroimaging Unit at INSERM in France**.

How Sleep Deprivation Sets You Back

When you're working on improving your inner AI, refining your habits, thought patterns, energy management, every day matters. A poor night's sleep doesn't just leave you tired. It skews perception, lowers resilience, amplifies negative thinking loops, and makes you more likely to abandon the progress you've made in rewiring limiting beliefs.

It's also why decisions made after long hours or poor sleep tend to be reactive, not strategic. In business, relationships, fitness, or personal growth, you cannot afford to operate with a compromised mind. The negative momentum from poor sleep can linger for days, subtly derailing your trajectory.

A Simple New Rule to Power Your AI

Commit to protecting your sleep like you protect your most valuable asset, because it is. Aim for **7–8 hours of quality sleep**, with consistent sleeping and waking times. Track how your thoughts, focus, and motivation shift when you prioritise rest.

Use the quiet moment before sleep to reinforce a thought or intention you want your subconscious to work on while you rest. Your AI is always listening, especially when conscious noise is turned down.

Remember:

A rested mind doesn't just think better. It chooses better, it feels better, and it sees opportunities that a fatigued mind will miss.

The Stories We Tell — And the Names We Give

One of the greatest revelations you'll have on this journey is realising just how much of your reality is shaped by the stories you tell yourself.

Your mind is constantly listening. It listens when you complain. It listens when you excuse. It listens when you label a feeling, a setback, or a symptom, and once you name it, **you give it identity, shape, and often power over you.**

We live in a world obsessed with naming conditions. Feeling exhausted? It's "burnout."

Anxious? It's "high-functioning anxiety." Can't focus? Maybe it's "adult ADHD."

Your back hurts? Must be "chronic lower lumbar dysfunction."

Now — is naming something always bad? No. Awareness matters. But **the danger lies in what happens next.**

Once named, we often **feed it, wear it like a badge, and unconsciously energise it.** The story becomes a part of our identity. The mind, your Original AI, then runs this narrative as a program, reinforcing it through every thought, word, and conversation you have about it.

And here's the problem: **the mind feeds on the stories we tell it.**

If you repeat a story of limitation, it runs a limitation program.

If you repeat a story of resilience and recovery, it runs a resilience program.

Your AI isn't judging. It's obeying.

It doesn't decide what's good or bad for you, it simply follows the dominant instruction.

And so what happens?

The false feed of disempowering information, the mental obsession with labels, conditions, and complaints, **creates unease in the body, and unease left unchecked becomes disease.** That stiff neck you keep calling a "recurring problem" becomes precisely that, not because your body can't heal, but because your AI has been ordered to hold onto it, keep looking for it, and give it meaning.

But the moment you consciously choose to stop energizing what no longer serves you, **everything begins to shift.**

You'll be amazed at how quickly symptoms begin to ease, not because you've ignored them, but because you've removed the constant instruction to focus on them.

This is the real power you've had all along.

The power to command your AI, to feed it with conscious stories of healing, strength, clarity, and recovery. To name not your limitations, but your victories, your progress, and your commitment to living with energy and intent.

From today, be hyper-aware of the labels you're carrying. Question whether they serve you.

And if they don't, drop them.

Tell a better story. Write a new script.

And watch how quickly your mind and body respond.

Universal Energies — The Invisible Flow That Shapes Us

Let's pause and remember what this book is really about: empowerment.

The words on these pages aren't here to tell you what to think, they're here to trigger what's already inside you, waiting to be awakened.

One of the greatest truths we can realise is that **we are constantly moving through a sea of energy**. Every person, every place, every thought carries its own frequency, and as we move through life, we cross paths with these energies. Some lift us. Some challenge us. Some leave an invisible mark we carry without realising it.

The powerful shift comes when you develop the awareness to feel it.

When you start to notice how you feel in different rooms, around certain people, in specific environments, you realise you're not just moving through life; you're moving through fields of influence. And with every encounter, a thought is created, a decision is made, a potential program is either added to your AI… or rejected.

The real mastery is in the pause.

When something doesn't align with the version of you you're working to build, stop. Breathe. Recognise it. You don't have to absorb every frequency you come into contact with. You get to choose what stays and what passes.

It's no accident you've felt it before, the shift in the room when someone walks in. The undeniable weight or lightness of their presence. And they've felt yours too. **That's energy. That's unspoken intelligence. That's the original AI at work.**

From now on, make a conscious decision to tune in.

Use every interaction as an opportunity to power up, to learn, to filter what belongs in your system and what doesn't. Not everyone will move to your rhythm. And that's okay. The goal isn't to control the energies around you, but to master how you respond within them.

This is a superpower.

Once you claim it, you'll no longer be unconsciously shaped by the world, you'll be shaping your world from within.

And that's how you begin to fuel your AI mind with clarity, strength, and purpose.

The Engine Room — How Your Mind Runs the Show

Before we can train and strengthen the mind, we need to understand how it operates day to day. Imagine your brain like a powerful operating system running behind the scenes, constantly scanning, adjusting, and managing every part of your body, whether you're aware of it or not.

Picture a pie chart representing **100% of your brain's daily activity**.

A significant percentage is dedicated to monitoring your vital organs: your heart, lungs, kidneys, digestive system, immune responses, and even itself, the brain. Another chunk is constantly scanning for problems to fix: repairing tissues, managing hormone levels, regulating blood pressure, and ensuring you stay alive and functional.

And here's the part most people never consider:

All of this consumes energy.

Not the kind you get by plugging into a wall socket, but the fuel you put into your body every single day. The quality of that fuel determines how efficiently your body and mind operate. Think of it like this, put low-grade, dirty fuel into a high-performance car, and it will cough, splutter, lose power, and underperform. Put in clean, high-octane fuel, and it runs smooth, powerful, and precise.

Your body is no different.

Poor nutrition forces your system to work harder to process and break down bad fuel, processed, artificial, chemical-laden food, stealing valuable energy away from the brain's primary functions. Energy that should be reserved for higher thinking, emotional regulation, clarity, and progress gets rerouted to cleaning up internal messes.

And now, add to that the constant demands on your mind to deal with old subconscious programs, unresolved emotions, and limiting beliefs. It's no wonder so many people feel mentally foggy, emotionally drained, and physically exhausted.

Here's the simple truth:

When your body is fed well, it recovers better. When it recovers better, your brain has the energy it needs to operate cleanly and powerfully. And when your mind is running clear, you are finally in a position to make the changes you desire, handle setbacks with resilience, and move towards the life you want with purpose.

This book is about training the mind and fuelling the body, because **both need to work together for you to perform at your best. Your mind is your original AI. Your body is the vehicle it drives. Fuel them both well, and you won't just survive, you'll thrive.**

Exercise — Demanding on the Body, Powerful for the Mind

Exercise isn't just something we do to look better or get fit, it's a powerful tool that directly affects the way our mind functions, processes information, and recovers. In fact, when you look at how much demand it places on both body and brain, it becomes clear that exercise isn't just physical, it's a mental game too.

Let's break it down.

Energy Demand during Exercise

When you exercise, you're asking your body to use more energy than it typically would during rest.

Refer back to the "pie" of brain function we spoke about earlier. A portion of your daily energy is already committed to vital body functions, heart, lungs, digestion, tissue repair, immune function, and subconscious programming. Now, introduce exercise and you're slicing off another piece of that energy pie to fuel movement: muscle contraction, oxygen distribution, heat regulation, and mental focus to maintain form, rhythm, and awareness.

The more intense or longer the exercise, the more energy it requires, not just physically, but mentally. This is why after a heavy workout or run, you often feel mentally drained too.

Recovery — The Other Half of the Story

What most people forget is that the real benefits of exercise don't happen while you're working out, they happen **during recovery**.

Your body needs time and the right resources (nutrients, hydration, sleep) to repair muscle tissue, replenish energy stores, and restore balance.

And this takes even more energy.

So now, even after your workout is done, your brain is still allocating extra energy to manage the recovery process: sending signals to repair muscle fibres, regulate inflammation, process waste byproducts like lactic acid, and return your system to homeostasis.

Without proper recovery, your mind stays stuck in a fatigued state, physically and mentally, which can lead to frustration, mood swings, and poor decision-making.

Exercise Goals — One Size Doesn't Fit All

Another key point: exercise is not a one-size-fits-all.

Some of us are aiming for high performance, perhaps a marathon, triathlon, or even Olympic-level ambitions. Others are doing it for general health, stress relief, or the satisfaction of completing a 10k fun run.

Then there's bodybuilding.

This isn't just about lifting weights. It's an entirely different level of discipline, nutrition, recovery, and mental focus. The brain's energy pie gets even more divided here, not only fuelling intense physical sessions but managing constant nutritional intake, sleep cycles, and mindset discipline to push through mental and physical barriers daily.

Whatever your goal is, it's important to recognise that **exercise is more demanding on your mind and body than most people give it credit for**. And with those demands come great rewards, but only when you support it properly.

The truth is, most people are operating inefficiently.

We're running outdated programs, carrying unhelpful beliefs, fueling our bodies with poor nutrition, and ignoring the natural positive energies around us that can actually help us reset and recharge.

Let's simplify this.

Imagine your body like a power grid.

A percentage of your daily energy goes toward running vital functions: your heart, lungs, brain, digestion, and subconscious scanning for problems and imbalances. That alone is a constant, heavy load. Then we add exercise, a wonderful, essential activity, but one that demands energy both to perform and to recover from.

But here's where the disconnect happens.

If you're carrying outdated beliefs, negative thought loops, poor nutrition, and ignoring your environment's energy, your system runs clunky. Like an old computer operating on too many background processes, everything slows down. The result?

Exhaustion, poor recovery, mental fog, tension, and injuries that linger.

Now factor in age. A teenager's system is still developing, awakening muscles, tendons, bones, and neurons. Their energy demands are high, but their recovery is faster because the body's natural growth phase is already on overdrive.

In our 20s and 30s, the body still handles strain well, muscle mass is easier to maintain, hormone levels support recovery, and mental resilience is naturally sharper.

Then in our 40s, 50s and beyond, lifestyle, accumulated stress, declining hormones, and entrenched beliefs start to show. The natural tendency is for recovery to slow and for energy systems to become less efficient. But it isn't because the body can't perform — it's often because the *mind and energy system aren't working in sync.*

And this is where we reclaim control.

It starts with reconnecting.

Movement is medicine, not just physically, but energetically. Exercise isn't just about burning calories or building muscle, it's a way to **realign your internal energy and reconnect with the positive, natural forces outside of you**.

A walk on the beach. A run as the sun rises. Stretching under trees. Breathing in open air.

Science backs this too, movement in nature improves serotonin, lowers cortisol, and regulates nervous system responses. It's the original energy recharge. And when combined with positive self-talk, clear nutrition, and conscious recovery, the body begins to shift from sluggish, disconnected survival mode to fluid, efficient, thriving mode.

Let me share Big Kev's story again, but from another angle.

Kev was carrying not just extra weight, but years of subconscious identity as *the big bloke*. He wore it like armor. As the kilos dropped and his fitness improved, an invisible tension crept in — not from his muscles, but from his mind's fear of becoming someone different. The result? His recovery slowed. Progress stalled. Injuries lingered.

It wasn't until we aligned his mind with his goal — shedding not just weight, but outdated beliefs — and started moving outdoors, focusing on gratitude, and consciously breathing in positive energy from his environment, that everything changed. His system synced up. The old programs cleared. Progress felt easier.

The lesson is simple but powerful:

Your energy isn't just fuel, it's information. It's connection. It's flow. When you move your body, clean your nutrition, calm your mind, and open yourself to the positive forces around you, you plug into a power source far greater than your own.

Your performance lifts. Recovery improves. Mental clarity sharpens. And life itself feels lighter.

"The mind and body are not separate. What affects one, affects the other. What heals one, heals them both."

So now, let's get you reconnected, cleared out, and tuned up. You're not here to just exist.

You're here to move, feel, and thrive.

Why It Matters

Understanding this allows you to plan better. You'll know when to push, when to recover, and when to adjust your nutrition to meet your activity level.

You'll also become more aware of how **mental fatigue affects your decisions and performance**, both inside the gym and out in the real world.

Movement is medicine for the mind. But like any medicine, it requires the right dose, the right timing, and the right recovery.

Later in the book, we'll go deeper into training types, how different demands affect your internal AI, and how to program your training to work with your body, not against it.

For now, remember this:

The more demands you place on your system, the more intentional

you must be about fuelling and recharging it. Exercise isn't just about sweating, it's about upgrading the mind-body system you live in.

Let me share another story, an experience with another client.

The Story of Sarah — And the Power from it.

I want to share this story for two reasons: for those who train, wanting to improve their body and fitness, and for those working to strengthen their inner AI, the mind within. Because the process is the same.

Sarah approached me while I was training a client. She quietly asked for a business card, which, at the time, I didn't have. I told her I wouldn't be long, and asked where she'd be. "The cardio machine," she replied.

When we finally sat down to talk, it quickly became clear that she wasn't entirely sure what she wanted. I could sense it in her posture: shoulders rolled forward, the energy of someone hiding from the world. She carried weight on her legs, what I saw as baby fat she'd never let go of, and she lacked confidence in her body, particularly in her upper frame.

I gave her a suggestion based on what I felt she was asking for but couldn't express: *"We need to trim those legs down, and we need to get you standing tall, shoulders back, with presence."* I told her I needed 12 weeks, and her full commitment to a program focused on building lean muscle to burn fat. And I warned her honestly: *"You'll feel bigger before you feel better. But trust me, it's part of the process."*

To Sarah's credit, she showed up every week. She stuck to the eating plan I set for her. Around week 10, she looked at me and said, *"Are you sure this is working? I feel heavier than when I started."*

I reminded her, *"Trust the process. We're close."*

By week 13, Sarah walked into the gym glowing. *"What happened?"* she asked. *"This is incredible. I can't believe how many compliments I've had. I feel amazing."*

Why do I share this story? Because life works exactly the same way.

Whether you're chasing a fitness goal or building the upgraded version of yourself through this AI work, it's a compounding effect. You won't always see the changes day to day. There will be moments of doubt, discomfort, and frustration. But those small daily investments, those little actions, add up. Until one day, you walk into your world, and people feel it. *You feel it.*

And in that moment, you realise, every uncomfortable step was worth it.

It takes time, trust, and consistency. But it's working, even when you don't yet see it.

The Box Story — Your Inner Sanctuary

Let me leave you with one of the most important ideas I've learned on this journey.

It's simple, but if you understand it, it'll change the way you move through your world.

We all crave a sense of safety — a constant we can rely on.

Think of a child with their security blanket or favourite toy. That child, born with all the natural powers of love, courage, curiosity, joy and truth, heads out into the world, plays, explores, stumbles, learns. But at some point, they return to that blanket, to recalibrate, to feel safe, to process it all. That moment of reassurance is how they prepare to head back out and do it all again.

Now here's the thing — as adults, we don't lose that need.

We might swap the blanket for a compliment, a relationship, a job title, a number in our bank account, or some external validation. When we get it, it fuels us, reassures us, says *"you're okay, keep going."* The problem is, we keep depending on things outside ourselves to give us that power.

What I want for you, and what this book and its teachings are really about, is building that security from within.

Here's how I explain it to myself — The Box Story.

Picture yourself inside a box.

The walls of this box are your protective shield, your beliefs, your habits, your comfort zone. You live from inside this box because it feels safe. Life happens outside the box, and sometimes you see something you want, or you get challenged, or an opportunity arrives, and you have to step outside those walls to grow.
That's natural.

But after you experience something new, a success, a failure, a moment of uncertainty, you instinctively retreat back into your box. The question is: *how long do you stay out of alignment before finding your grounding again?*

The goal isn't to never leave the box.

It's to make the return quicker and stronger each time.

To know you have a place within yourself, an unshakeable, self-powered security system, where you can pause, reflect, recalibrate, and then step back out with greater awareness and confidence.

The better you get at this, the less you rely on the world to give you validation or reassurance. You begin to generate your own energy, your own certainty. **You become your own security blanket.**

That's what strengthens your AI, your internal operating system.

Because when you realise you can consciously notice when you've stepped off track, pause, breathe, anchor yourself back to your true values and intentions, and return to action, you've mastered one of the greatest powers available to you as a human being.

This is what I want for you.

A mind so tuned in to its own energy and worth, that external opinions, setbacks, and temporary discomfort don't throw you off for long.

A system where you become your own managing director, guiding your life's momentum through conscious awareness and choice.

That's the real security we've been searching for. And it's always been inside you.

"Validation is addictive. Inner certainty is unstoppable."

"Own your story, or you'll get lost in someone else's version of it."
"Your energy is currency. Don't spend it on cheap opinions."

Now, get to work, build your awareness, sharpen your AI, and create the life you know you're capable of living.

The Power of Cold Showers: Building Awareness, Resilience, and a Sharper Mind

It's no secret that cold plunges and ice baths have exploded in popularity. Wellness influencers, elite athletes, and biohackers alike swear by their benefits, from improved recovery to mental clarity and stress resilience. But you don't need a membership to a fancy wellness centre to access these benefits. In fact, one of the most effective tools for building awareness, mental toughness, and body control is sitting right in your own home: your shower.

Yes — the cold shower.

Most people recoil at the thought, and that's exactly why it's powerful. The simple act of choosing discomfort, even briefly, is a training ground for your willpower and self- awareness. Each second you stand under cold water, you override your mind's default wiring that's conditioned to avoid discomfort. This is your moment of decision, your personal laboratory to observe how your mind responds when faced with challenge, and how you can rewire it.

Why Cold Showers? What Happens to the Body and Mind

When exposed to cold water, your blood vessels constrict, your heart rate elevates, and your nervous system instantly switches to a heightened state. Endorphins are released, inflammation is reduced, circulation improves, and stress hormones begin to regulate. But what's often overlooked is what happens to your **mind**.

A cold shower triggers a flood of immediate, primal thoughts: *"Get out!"* *"This is unbearable!"* *"Why are you doing this?"* That's your subconscious programming fighting for control. This is precisely where the power lies, not in enduring the cold, but in observing these reactions and consciously choosing your response. It sharpens your internal AI's ability to stay composed under pressure, to make clear decisions amid discomfort, and to expand the threshold of what you believe you can handle.

A Practical, Simple Way to Start

You don't need to start with full-minute ice baths. A practical, mindful way to introduce this into your routine is by using the wait time at the start of your shower. While waiting for the water to warm up, turn it to cold and step in. Even 10–15 seconds is enough to trigger the response. Focus on your breathing, deep, steady, nose breathing if possible, and consciously acknowledge the discomfort without reacting. This is your daily ritual of control.

Each day, add 5–10 seconds. Not as a punishment, but as a commitment to growth. As the days pass, you'll notice not just physical benefits like increased energy and sharper alertness, but also a calmer mind when life throws the unexpected at you.

Use This Time Wisely

This brief cold exposure isn't just a physical act — it's an opportunity for reflection. Use those seconds to run through empowering thoughts:

- "I am stronger than this moment."

- "Discomfort is my training ground."

- "This is sharpening my awareness."

- "I decide how I feel, not my circumstances."

You're no longer waiting for your shower to warm up, you're actively warming up your mind to handle life.

The Bigger Picture

Small acts of conscious discomfort build resilience. They teach you that you can act despite resistance, that your AI is trainable, and that your willpower is a muscle. In a world engineered for comfort, those who master discomfort gain the edge.

And remember, cold showers aren't just a health hack, they're a daily reminder that you are in charge of your mind, your energy, and your responses.

"Discomfort is not your enemy — it's the doorway to your next level of strength, clarity, and control."

The Invisible Trap of Old Wives' Tales: How Belief Becomes Biology

If there's one thing I need you to truly absorb from this chapter, it's this: **what we believe, we invite into our reality.** Not just emotionally, but physically, chemically, and energetically. And nothing illustrates this better than the stories and superstitions we absorb from others without questioning.

Let me explain through a real story from my years of personal training.

Client Story: The 'Cold Wind' Curse

I once had a strong, no-nonsense client. Driven, intense, with a fierce need to control and understand every aspect of her training and body. That kind of focus can be a strength if channelled well, but here's where it got interesting.

She would tell me, *"I had the back of my neck exposed to a cold wind while sitting at a café — I'm going to get sick, I know it."*

Sure enough, within 24 hours, she'd fall ill. It happened once, twice, then again. Always the same trigger, always the same outcome.

I started to pay attention. She later revealed this pattern had followed her for years, on holidays, at events, at family gatherings.

If a breeze hit the back of her neck, she'd *predict illness*, and her body would oblige. Now, here's the frighteningly powerful part.

This was never about the cold wind. It was about the story.

A belief system so deeply embedded, likely passed down generationally as an old wives' tale, that it operated as a program within her subconscious AI. The conviction of her expectation — *I will get sick now* — was so strong, her body adapted to match it.

Think about what that means.

We have that much power to turn belief into biology.

Not always consciously, but through subconscious programs absorbed from family, culture, or past experience.

Now imagine if that same energy was directed at something useful.

What if she'd said: *"My lower back's tight, but I'll wake up pain-free tomorrow."*

Or: *"Today I'll feel stronger and sharper with every step I take."*

That's how powerful our AI is. It responds to **repeated instruction delivered with conviction,** whether helpful or harmful.

Why This Is Dangerous: The 'I Was Right' Trap

And here's the deeper issue.

When her prediction came true, she wasn't disappointed.

She was satisfied.

Why? Because we take comfort in being right. It reinforces the sense of control, even if the outcome is negative.

That subtle validation — *"See? I knew it."* — becomes a reward in the subconscious mind. It strengthens a program that limits us. And it happens everywhere:

- *I knew I'd hate that event.*
- *I knew they'd let me down.*
- *I knew I'd mess this up.*

Being right feeds our false beliefs.

It provides a sense of security, even when it keeps us trapped in low-grade outcomes.

Over time, this leads to what I call *chronic prediction mode* — where we constantly anticipate outcomes just to be proven right. And since no one can predict life perfectly, this eventually results in disappointment, eroded motivation, and an AI operating off limited data and outdated programs.

Your Challenge: Where Are You Predicting Yourself?

Now here's your work:

- **Where in your life are you making predictions just to be right?**
- **What old sayings, beliefs, or superstitions have you inherited that shape how you interpret events?**
- **How often do you pre-empt outcomes just so you can say, "See, I knew it" — even when it harms you?**

Recognising this is powerful.

It's another way to stay mindful, and it's a tool for rewriting the faulty code in your subconscious AI.

The goal is not to stop thinking ahead, but to ensure your predictions are **empowering, expansive, and aligned with the outcomes you actually want.**

Because belief, repeated, turns into biology. And you get to choose what you believe.

Ok — here you go. I'll give you a couple of examples to get you started.

Example 1: Business

Ever caught yourself thinking *"This meeting's going to be a waste of time"* before it even started?

And then, you show up distracted, half-engaged, and surprise surprise, it was a waste of time.

Not because it had to be, but because your energy shaped it that way.

Example 2: Relationships

How about that moment before a social event when you tell yourself *"No one will really care that I'm there"* — so you arrive guarded, detached, and don't let people in.

And you leave convinced you were right, when in fact you never gave them the chance.

Example 3: Health

You wake up feeling a little off, and instantly tell yourself *"I'm getting sick — I always catch something this time of year."*

From that moment on, your mind scans for proof: a sniffle here, a slight ache there. You slow down, expect it, and your body obliges.

The belief shapes the biology.

Not because the sniffle was dangerous — but because the thought became a command your AI obeyed.

Example 4: Self-Image

Ever looked in the mirror and thought *"I've always had terrible shoulders"* or *"I'll never be one of those people who looks confident"*?

And so when you walk into a room, your posture follows the prediction. You shrink a little, avoid eye contact, and reinforce the very belief you'd hoped to escape.

The mind wrote the program, and the body followed it.

Now, your challenge still stands:

Where else in your life are you making these invisible predictions, and living them out like a script?

Find them and when you do, don't get frustrated.

Smile, because you've just found the lever to change your AI.

This isn't about blame. It's about power.

Because if you can find them, you can change them.

And with each one you dismantle, you sharpen your AI and reclaim your future.

"The stories we tell ourselves aren't harmless — they're blueprints the body builds from, and futures the mind walks into."

Training Hurdles, Niggles, and The Power of Conscious Control

One of the most valuable discoveries I've made in both my own training and coaching others is how often those daily niggles, the little aches, tight spots, or stubborn pains, aren't just physical issues, but signs of congestion in our internal energy flow. Left unchecked, they become anchors that slow our system down. And while we've been conditioned to either ignore them or hand them off for someone else to fix, those signals are opportunities.

When you begin to operate with conscious awareness, you realise these niggles are not inconveniences, they're feedback. The body is asking for attention, for recalibration. And when you start to truly work with this awareness, you're strengthening your AI, refining your system's ability to detect, respond, and self-correct.

Here's the process I've found most powerful:

The moment you notice discomfort, don't dismiss it. Stop, breathe, and consciously direct your attention into that area. The act of slowing down, checking in with yourself, and mentally connecting to where it hurts or feels tight does more than you might imagine. It disrupts the automated 'ignore and push through' program most of us run daily.

Once you've acknowledged the signal, stretch the area. But stretch it with intention. Don't go through the motions. Stay connected to that spot. Notice how it feels, how it responds. You'll find most minor issues begin to ease simply because you brought awareness and energy flow to them.

And here's the deeper power: each time you take ownership of a niggle, rather than outsourcing it, you're not just fixing a physical problem, you're upgrading your mind-body operating system. You're sharpening your internal AI's responsiveness. Over time, this cultivates a mind and body more in sync, more resilient, and better able to avoid bigger issues before they happen.

Of course, if something persists, always seek professional help, but do so with the knowledge that your own efforts will make their work more effective. You'll heal faster, your practitioner will notice the difference, and you'll walk away not just fixed, but empowered.

This is the kind of mastery we're building here: one where you no longer live at the mercy of your body's setbacks, but instead use every challenge as another opportunity to deepen your awareness, sharpen your mind-body connection, and strengthen the original AI that is you.

Cutting Through the Noise — Taking Back Control

As we mentioned in *Mind: The Original AI*, none of us came into this world with an instruction manual. From the moment we arrive, we're left to figure out how to operate this incredible system, the mind, the body, our emotions, our energy, nutrition, sleep, all while being thrown into an environment that rarely slows down long enough for us to make sense of it and if that wasn't enough, on top of that comes the constant bombardment.

Open any health magazine or scroll through your phone, and you'll find conflicting advice at every turn. "This is the best diet." "That's the workout program you need." "Here's how you can get the perfect body in six weeks." It's exhausting, and more importantly, it's confusing. One message after another designed to sell you something, often without real consideration for what you actually need.

This book, and this next stage of your journey, is about cutting through that noise.

The difference now is, you've started programming your own operating system. You're no longer approaching life's choices blindly or reacting to every new trend. You've built awareness. You're becoming conscious of how your thoughts, habits, and energy work together.

Now, when a new diet fad comes along, instead of being pulled by it, you'll ask:

"Is this right for me? Does this serve my goals, my health, my body?"

When a flashy fitness challenge appears, you'll check in:

"Does this align with my plan? Is this adding value or just adding noise?"

This section, and this book, is about taking back control.

It's about learning to recognise information for what it is: **options**, not orders.

You'll start filtering through advice, opinions, and trends using your own upgraded, personal operating system.

And here's the best part: you'll finally stop wasting energy chasing what was never designed for you, and start focusing on what genuinely improves your life.

From here, we'll sharpen this system even more, so you can move through the world clearer, lighter, and with your own roadmap.

The Body's Goal — And It's Not What You Think

Let's go deeper. It's time to get properly acquainted with this remarkable vehicle you live in, your body. And here's something most people never realise:

The body has its own goal.

When I was working as a fitness coach, one of the first things I'd ask clients was, *"What's your goal?"*

I'd hear the usual: *"I want to lose weight." "I want to be healthier." "I want to look good for summer."*

Then I'd ask, *"Do you know what your body's goal is?"*

And not one of them ever got it right.

The body's only real goal is to stay alive.

That's it.

It doesn't care about your dream car, your perfect partner, your beach holiday, or whether you feel emotionally balanced. Its job, its entire operating system, is designed around one single outcome: survival.

And here's where it gets interesting.

Because the body is so good at adapting and keeping you alive, it tolerates the punishment you give it. Late nights, junk food, stress, lack of movement, toxins, negative thoughts, and yet you wake up the next day. You're still breathing. And because you survived, the subconscious mind records that experience as *acceptable*.

"See? We made it. You're still here."

But the question we rarely ask is, *at what cost?*

Every time you burn the candle at both ends, binge on rubbish food, let stress run your nervous system, or push through exhaustion, you may survive it… but you're also setting new baselines for your future. You're writing programs into your subconscious that say: **"This is normal. This is what we do."**

And that's the lie we keep feeding ourselves. *"I had a big night out, but I'm still alive." "I ate terrible food, but I made it through."*

Yes, the body got you through it, because that's its job. But inside, it's working overtime, re- routing energy, compensating, repairing, draining reserves you can't see, all while you tell yourself you're fine. This is the silent cost. And over time, it adds up.

The revelation here is that most people never stop to consider this. They never realise that survival isn't thriving.

They mistake the body's resilience for permission to keep mistreating it.

In this chapter, we're going to reset that relationship.

We'll start treating the body not as something that just gets dragged along for the ride, but as an intelligent, responsive system with its own priorities, and when you learn to work with it, rather than against it, everything in your life begins to shift.

This is your call to wake up from the illusion of "I'm still alive, so I must be okay." Because you deserve far better than just surviving.

Now — let's be clear.

This isn't about living like a monk, cutting out every pleasure, or avoiding every social moment. Life is meant to be experienced, enjoyed, and shared. Drinks with friends, a spontaneous meal on a busy day, an indulgent dessert, these aren't the problem.

The issue isn't the moment — it's the meaning we attach to it.

The real damage happens when we **layer those moments with guilt** and self-criticism. When you beat yourself up over a night out, a skipped workout, or grabbing takeaway on the run, you're not just punishing yourself emotionally, you're reinforcing negative patterns in the subconscious.

You're writing a program that says:
"I always fail."
"I can't stick to anything." "I'm not disciplined."

And over time, those beliefs shape how you feel, act, and show up in life.

The trick is to drop the guilt.

Enjoy life. Make room for it. Just don't let those moments rewrite your identity.

An old saying sums this up perfectly:

"Don't throw the baby out with the bathwater."

If you slip, if you stray, **simply get back on track.**

Contrast is part of the process.

The yin and yang, the ups and downs, they give you reference points.

Without challenge, you wouldn't appreciate ease. Without mistakes, you wouldn't learn.

So embrace the whole process.

Celebrate your wins, acknowledge the off days without judgment, and always return to your path.

That's how you reprogram your AI, with wisdom, not punishment.

Check points

You start to feel momentum, progress is happening. You're becoming more aware, pausing, adjusting, and moving with intention. But then… something slips. You find yourself off- track. A moment of doubt. A lapse in focus. What felt aligned now feels disconnected.

It's not failure. It's familiar patterns trying to reclaim their place, often at very specific times of the day.

Maybe it's the afternoon slump, when your energy dips and old habits try to sneak back in.

Maybe it's the evening, when "unwinding" becomes a quiet undoing of the progress you made.

Maybe its 3am, you wake up, and instead of calm, your mind begins the loop of doubt or distraction.

These are not signs you're going backwards. These are your checkpoints.

And now that you've identified them, they become power plays for serious change. Awareness is the beginning of mastery. The moment you see the pattern, you can shift it. The moment you pause, your inner intelligence kicks in.

That's the original AI, and it's working for you.

Life is already changing in response to your decision to change.Now, trust what you've created. Adjust with it. Own it.

Catching a Cold — The Body's Cleansing Process

Most people, when they start feeling sick, slip into frustration, self-pity, and a loss of motivation. But what if we completely flipped that mindset?

What if feeling under the weather was actually your body doing you a favour?

When you catch a cold, experience fatigue, or get hit with a bout of flu-like symptoms, it's not random. It's your system cleansing itself, working overtime to deal with the accumulated waste from poor nutrition, stagnant energy, unresolved stress, and subconscious tension.

Think about it: where do you imagine that 'gunk' comes from?

It isn't dumped on us by the outside world. It's the result of choices, the food we eat, the thoughts we carry, the unresolved emotions we store, and the energy we fail to clear. When the body reaches a tipping point, it triggers a clean-out.

That runny nose, sore throat, fever, and fatigue? That's your biological operating system processing and expelling what doesn't belong.

Reframe the Experience

Instead of letting sickness drag you down mentally, use it as a powerful reset:

- **Slow down.** Rest is essential, it's your AI recalibrating.

- **Hydrate and nourish.** Give your system clean fuel to assist the process.

- **Use the time to reflect.** Where have you been pushing too hard, neglecting yourself, or ignoring what your AI has been whispering?

- **Mentally thank your body.** It's working to keep you alive, no matter what you've thrown at it.

Build a Better Operating System

Here's the truth: every time you recover from being unwell, your AI and immune system upgrade — if you let it.

Use this time to reset your mindset, clear emotional clutter, and recommit to healthier habits. The real trick is to avoid falling into negative thought loops and instead choose to see illness as productive downtime, a necessary cleanse to stay sharp.

Every setback holds the seeds for your next level of growth.

Learn to recognise the process, and you'll be amazed at how quickly your recovery speeds up, both physically and mentally.

Fuel for the Original AI: How Nutrition Drives Mind and Body Efficiency

Food, as we all know, is essential for survival, but survival is not enough. **The real key to an energised, clear, and resilient life is not just the energy food provides, but the *quality of nutrition* it delivers.** And now that you've begun taking a more conscious, intentional approach to how you operate, it's time to look at how we can use food and nutrition with intelligence, to optimise outcomes for both your body and your mind.

Here's the foundation: **we are made up of protein, fat, carbohydrates, water, and minerals.**

And while fats, carbs, and water can be stored, **protein cannot.** Your muscles, organs, enzymes, hormones, and even neurotransmitters are built from protein, or more specifically, the amino acids protein is broken down into.

Why does this matter?

Because if your diet isn't consistently supplying the protein your body needs to regenerate cells, repair tissues, and build new structures, **the body will start to harvest it from your own muscle tissue.**

This is called **catabolism,** and over time, it contributes to muscle wasting, weakness, slower recovery, reduced metabolism, and even cognitive decline. What's worse, the body's survival instinct kicks in, slowing down vital processes to reduce demand for these amino acids, effectively putting your system into energy conservation mode.

Now add to this the load of old, inefficient subconscious programs you're carrying. The energy your brain allocates to daily maintenance, healing, thinking, and emotional regulation is already stretched. Poor nutrition only amplifies this inefficiency. The result is fatigue, foggy thinking, reduced motivation, and an AI (your mind) that starts working against you instead of for you.

The Science of Nutrition and Cognitive Performance

Multiple studies confirm that diets higher in quality protein, omega-3 fatty acids, vitamins B12, D, and antioxidants **improve memory, mood regulation, and cognitive function.** Poor dietary patterns, high in processed carbs, sugars, trans fats, and low nutrient density, have been directly linked to increased rates of depression, anxiety, and cognitive decline. **In short: the cleaner your fuel, the clearer your mind.**

My Most Effective Daily Energy Hack

One of the most powerful shifts I made for sustained energy, mental clarity, and emotional steadiness was changing how I woke my body up in the morning.

Here's the mistake most people make:

They wake up, but their body isn't truly *awake*. They immediately consume heavy, dense foods, bread, bacon, processed cereals, or worse, skip food entirely and rely on coffee. This is like trying to pour petrol on cold coals.

The smarter way is to light the furnace first.

Start your day with a small, light food that's easy to digest, a piece of fruit is ideal. It's high in natural sugars, water content, vitamins, and enzymes, providing an immediate, gentle wake-up call for your digestive system and metabolism.

Why?

Because your body needs a signal, like kindling for a fire.

Once the system is gently activated, **wait 10–15 minutes, then consume a clean, balanced meal with quality protein.** This way, the body is primed to digest, absorb, and utilise nutrients efficiently, rather than being overwhelmed by a heavy load on a cold system.

The fruit idea can be done throughout the day when hungry, before eating your meal, fire up the metabolism.

The result?

- Cleaner energy.
- Sharper mental focus.
- Improved emotional regulation.
- And a subconscious state primed for positive program rewriting.

This isn't superstition, it's physiology.

The gut-brain axis, a complex communication network between your digestive tract and your brain, plays a direct role in hormone regulation, immune response, and cognitive function.

When you start your day intelligently, you control this feedback loop, **fuelling your Original AI to operate as your most powerful, reliable ally.**

Bottom line:

You're not just eating to stay alive. You're eating to wake up, to move with clarity, to feel strong, and to train your mind to work *for you, not against you.*

The quality of your nutrition today is programming the efficiency of your mind tomorrow. **"Your body is the hardware. Your mind is the software. Nutrition is the power source."** Time to fuel it like you mean it.

Remember, we find what we are looking for, find what we want.

The First Rule of Change: Define the Outcome and Make It Matter

One of the most important, and often overlooked, principles for creating real, lasting change in our lives is this: **before anything shifts, you must be crystal clear on what you want the outcome to be.** Not a vague wish, not a half-hearted idea, a clear, powerful, deeply personal goal that means something to you.

Here's why this matters:

Every time we attempt to make a change, resistance will show up. Thoughts like *"this is too hard," "I don't have time," "what's the point,"* or *"maybe I'll start next week"* will come knocking. If the purpose behind your goal isn't strong enough, those excuses will win.

But when the reward, the outcome you're chasing, is deeply meaningful, when it excites you, challenges you, and makes you feel alive just thinking about it, something powerful happens:

The obstacles shrink, the doubts lose their grip, and your internal AI (your subconscious programming) begins to align with your new direction.

This isn't just a motivational idea, it's a process you can apply to anything in life:

- **Want to improve your health?** Get clear on what life looks and feels like when you're thriving.

- **Chasing a financial goal?** See beyond the numbers to what that money will allow you to do, become, or contribute.

- **Working on your mindset?** Envision what kind of person you're becoming as those new beliefs take hold.

The stronger and clearer the outcome, the easier it is to stay the course when life inevitably throws distractions and resistance your way.

And here's the part most people miss:

With every attempt you make, and every success you experience, no matter how small, something within you starts to shift. An inner confidence begins to grow. You start to realise *"I can do this. I've done it before, I'll do it again."*

Each win, each choice, each breakthrough becomes a deposit into your internal belief system, strengthening your AI's operating code and making the next effort feel a little more possible, a little more natural, and a little more powerful.

That's how momentum is built. That's how confidence is earned. And that's how lasting change takes hold.

Why Consistency Matters: Earning the Body's Trust

If there's one thing your body craves, it's **consistency**.

The human body is an incredibly intelligent, adaptive system, but it's constantly scanning for patterns. It wants to know: *can I trust this person to give me what I need?*

When your nutrition, movement, rest, and thoughts are erratic, your body goes into protection mode. It slows processes, stores energy, and holds onto inflammation and tension because it's unsure what's coming next. It's like a cautious employee working for a boss who changes their mind every day, defensive, reactive, and inefficient.

But when you start showing up consistently, eating clean, moving your body, fuelling your mind, and prioritising recovery, something powerful happens.

Your body starts to trust you.

It learns that it doesn't need to hold back, store excess fat "just in case," or slow down to protect itself from poor inputs. It can release energy more freely, heal faster, and support clearer, more stable mental performance.

Each day you repeat these good habits, you're not just getting healthier, you're strengthening a relationship of trust between your conscious self and your Original AI. And like any relationship built on trust, **it gets easier, stronger, and more efficient with time.**

Consistency isn't perfection, it's reliability.

Give your body and mind a reason to rely on you, and they'll reward you in ways you never expected.

Harnessing Discipline: Lessons from the Field to the Mind

We might not be professional athletes, but there's a powerful lesson in watching those who push themselves to the limits of human performance, and it's not just about physical ability. It's about **commitment, discipline, and the ability to stay connected to a purpose, even when the work is tough.**

Take someone like **Scott Pendlebury**, ex captain of the Collingwood Football Club. Every morning, Scott wakes up with a clear sense of what he's working toward. His days aren't driven by guesswork or mood. They're guided by a plan: a specific focus on fuelling his body efficiently, training with purpose, recovering properly, and making decisions that align with the long game, not just for his body, but for his mind.

And here's the key:

That discipline isn't just physical. It sharpens his internal AI, the subconscious decision- making system that operates behind the scenes in all of us. By consistently feeding it clear instructions and disciplined actions, Scott's AI learns to work in his favour, helping him instinctively make good choices under pressure, stay composed in high-stakes moments, and recover quickly from setbacks.

Now, you don't have to be an AFL captain to live this way.

You might already know someone in your own world who embodies this discipline. Maybe it's a business owner you admire, a community leader, or even a family member. The point is, we're surrounded by examples of what it looks like to show up with purpose and consistency.

And the exciting part is this:

You have that same potential. Every time you wake up and decide to move your body, make a better nutrition choice, sit in stillness, or breathe deeply through a stressful moment — you're not just getting through the day. You're reprogramming your AI. You're teaching it to prioritise clarity over chaos, discipline over distraction, progress over excuses.

This is how champions are built.

Not by talent alone, but by a thousand small, consistent decisions that compound over time.

The real question isn't whether you have what it takes — it's whether you'll choose to show up for yourself like those you admire.

Because when you do, something incredible happens:

your motivation sharpens, your resilience grows, and your inner AI begins to operate on a higher level — one that works for you, not against you.

This is how we build our edge.

Evening Rituals for Reset & Recovery

Your morning sets the tone for the day, but your evening anchors your nervous system, primes your subconscious, and determines the quality of your next day's focus. Introducing a mindful wind-down routine isn't about being rigid, it's about training your AI to know when to power down and heal.

Suggested Practices:

- 10-minute evening walk, phone-free.

- Light stretches while focusing on breath.

- Gratitude reflection: 3 things you appreciated from the day.

- Mentally releasing tension from areas that feel heavy or tight.

- Avoid screen-time 30 minutes before sleep; replace with reading or meditation.

The Benefit: Reduces subconscious stress loops, improves sleep quality, and allows your AI to sort and store positive neural connections overnight.

Micro-Mindfulness for Energy Management

Energy isn't just physical, it's emotional and mental currency. Tiny unnoticed leaks throughout your day deplete your reserves. Reclaim them through micro-mindfulness.

- Pause before entering a room or meeting. Take a slow breath.
- Name what emotion you're carrying right now.
- Before sending a message, ask: "What energy am I putting into this?"

The Benefit: Sharpens awareness, recalibrates your inner AI, and prevents accumulated overwhelm.

Energy Leak Inventory

Where in your life are you leaking energy unnecessarily? Make a list:

- Conversations you replay mentally.
- People you say yes to out of guilt.
- Habits that drain your motivation.
- Environments that don't nourish you.

Action: Spot one leak this week and resolve it. Reclaim that bandwidth for yourself.

Reframing Symptoms & Niggles

Your body isn't betraying you — it's communicating with you. Niggles, tightness, or feeling flat aren't inconveniences, they're instructions.

New View:

- That back pain = area asking for attention.
- That fatigue = reminder to check your inputs.

Action: Instead of ignoring or medicating, pause and dialogue with it: *"What do you need from me right now?"* Trust what rises.

The Compounding Habit Effect

No great life transformation comes from one moment. It's the compounded effect of small aligned actions.

Principle:

- 1% better each day = exponential improvement.
- Miss a day? Don't break the chain two days in a row.

Mindset: View your habits like drops filling a reservoir. At first it seems insignificant — until the day it overflows with power.

Future Mapping Exercise

Imagine 3 versions of you in 3 years:

- If you change nothing.
- If you make moderate positive changes.
- If you fully commit to your AI work, health and awareness practices. **Action:** Write them out. Let the emotional impact guide your present decisions. **Reframing Regret**

Regret isn't failure — it's data. It shows you where your values and actions were misaligned.

New Script: Instead of *"I should have"* ☐ *"Now I know what matters to me."*

This turns past pain into a sharpening tool for your AI, rather than a weight you carry.

Upgrading Self-Talk Scripts

Your internal dialogue is a command line for your subconscious AI.

From:

- "I can't stick to anything." **To:**
- "I'm learning to honour my commitments."

From:

- "This always happens to me." **To:**
- "I'm creating a new pattern with each decision."

Daily Practice: Catch 3 negative phrases. Replace them immediately. Log them if needed.

The Power of a Grateful Pause

Modern neuroscience is starting to catch up with what ancient wisdom has always known — that the state of mind we enter *before* an action directly shapes the biological and energetic outcome of that action.

Studies in neurobiology and contemplative science have shown that a simple practice of gratitude or intention-setting before a meal, before exercise, even before a conversation, alters the neurochemical environment in your brain and body. It reduces stress markers, improves digestion, balances heart rate variability, and even enhances immune response.

But let's look deeper.

This isn't just about feeling good, it's about **priming your internal AI**.

Your subconscious, your personal, built-in AI, is constantly scanning your environment for cues to decide what programs to run. When you take a moment to pause before eating and silently acknowledge the food, its source, and the nourishment it offers, you send a signal to your AI:

"This moment matters. I am in control. I choose to nourish."

That signal doesn't just affect your meal, it rewires how your subconscious processes stress, relationships, and daily challenges.

It builds a pattern of awareness, and with consistency, creates a mental and energetic baseline of control and gratitude that influences everything you do.

And this can be done with anything:

- Before you train, give thanks for the body you have, even with its aches and niggles.
- Before you speak with someone, acknowledge the value of the connection, whether pleasant or difficult.
- Before you tackle a tough task, be grateful for the opportunity to grow stronger through it.

Every grateful pause is a command sent to your AI to work in your favour. It's a way of strengthening the signal that you run this system, not the noise of old programs, fears or automatic reactions.

And over time, these small moments stack up.

Not only will your health improve, but so will the quality of your thinking, your choices, and your ability to stay grounded amidst the chaos of life.

The greatest upgrade you can give your AI isn't a dramatic life change — it's hundreds of tiny, intentional moments where you choose to lead it.

Technology — Your Ally or Adversary?

In the age we live in, technology isn't just a tool — it's a force shaping how we think, move, connect, and even perceive ourselves. As much as it can enhance the quality of our lives, it can just as easily dull our instincts, distract our attention, and disconnect us from our internal power. The difference lies in how consciously we choose to engage with it.

This chapter isn't about abandoning technology — it's about reclaiming our position as its master, not its servant. **When approached mindfully, technology can become one of your greatest allies in strengthening your AI and navigating your personal evolution.**

Harnessing Technology to Sharpen the Process

We're surrounded by technology — in our homes, our pockets, our workplaces, and soon, as personal AI assistants and robots embedded in daily life. It's no longer a question of whether we'll use technology, but **how we'll use it**.

The risk is clear: if we allow ourselves to become too reliant, we outsource not just the doing, but the thinking. And that subtle shift, over time, begins to erode our personal agency, our sharpness, and our ability to self-direct.

But if used with intention, technology can offer incredible advantages:

- **It can provide contrast.** Like meditation or breathwork, the mindful use of a podcast, a playlist, or even a five-minute game can interrupt negative thought loops or fatigue, giving you a chance to reset.

- **It can streamline your systems.** Habit trackers, gratitude journals, AI scheduling tools — all of these can remove friction, allowing you to operate from clarity, not chaos.

- **It can amplify your growth.** With a world of books, lectures, guided sessions, and tools at your fingertips, self-education and AI strengthening have never been so accessible.

The trick is **to stay conscious**. Be the one deciding when, why, and how technology enters your day. Ask yourself: *Is this sharpening me, or sedating me?* Am I engaging with this to elevate my process — or avoid it?

The greatest danger isn't technology itself — it's unconscious use.

When you let it run on autopilot, it chips away at your awareness, your drive, your natural rhythms. But when you control it, when you position it as a tool in service of your personal evolution, it becomes a powerful amplifier of your AI and your life.

As a simple practice:

- Use tech for inspiration, learning, or measured contrast.
- Avoid mindless consumption.
- Make space for tech-free moments daily to keep your internal guidance system sharp.

In the end, technology isn't the enemy of your AI — unconscious use is.

Stay mindful, and turn your tech into a superpower.

Take the Helm — You Are the CEO of You

As you turn these final pages, I want to remind you of something important: **this book was never about giving you a set of strict rules or a one-size-fits-all plan.**

It was about handing you the keys to the most advanced operating system you will ever possess, **your mind. Your Original AI.**

In **Book One**, you discovered how your mind functions as an organic AI system, running on subconscious programs, old beliefs and learned patterns. You learned how to recognise those faulty codes, how to pause, reprogram and consciously install new, empowering beliefs. You learned the power of your thoughts, emotions, and how to reclaim command of your own inner dialogue.

Then in **Book Two**, we fuelled that AI.

We explored how the body, this incredible, self-regulating machine you've been gifted, responds to nutrition, exercise, breath, sleep, and emotional energy. We talked about how each choice you make either empowers your Original AI or clogs its system. You saw how clean fuel, intentional movement, and connected breathing don't just improve your physical health, they sharpen your mind and elevate your life experience.

And now, standing at this point in your journey, the message is simple:

You are the Managing Director. You are the CEO of You.

Your mind, body, energy, thoughts, habits, emotions, nutrition, sleep, and breath, these are the departments under your leadership. And just like a skilled CEO stepping into a new role, **you don't overhaul everything at once.**

You observe. You assess. You learn where the weaknesses are, where the untapped strengths live, and what adjustments will create the biggest impact.

You are no longer a passenger. You are no longer operating unconsciously.

The old programs you uncovered in Book One? You now have the awareness and the tools to rewrite them.

The habits you uncovered in Book Two? You now know how to nourish, move, and breathe in a way that sustains energy, sharpens clarity, and unlocks consistency.

This is where it all comes together.

Your job from here is to step into this leadership role with the quiet confidence of someone who understands the value of patience, awareness, and intelligent action.

Your AI is no longer running you. You're running it.

And the beautiful part? **You get to decide what happens next.**

You don't need to be perfect. You need to be present, tuned in, and willing to steer your life by conscious design.

So as you close this book, know this isn't an ending, it's the moment you assume command. **Lead yourself with wisdom. Train your AI daily. Fuel it with intention. Make your next chapter your finest yet.**

The helm is yours. Now, take it.

Every day, you're given a finite amount of energy, and how you choose to use it shapes the course of your life. When that energy is spent worrying — about things beyond your control or outcomes that haven't even happened — you slowly drain your strength, your focus, and your presence.

Worry is a thief.

It steals your clarity, your time, and your inner peace.

But here's the truth: the same energy used to fuel worry can be redirected, into vision, into resilience, into hope.

What we focus on expands.

If your thoughts are anchored in fear, doubt, and negativity, your life will reflect more of the same. But if you shift your focus, if you choose to see the opportunity within the obstacle, the growth within the struggle, you awaken the leader within.

Positivity isn't about pretending everything's fine. It's about choosing how you respond.

It's deciding that whatever stands before you, you will meet it with strength, clarity, and conviction.

Your mind is trainable, just like your body.

And training takes discipline. Be intentional with your thoughts. Guard your mindset like a leader guards their mission. Feed it with gratitude, with vision, with belief.

Because when you shift your thinking, you don't just change your mood, you change your momentum.

And momentum attracts progress, growth, and people who are ready to rise with you.

Periodisation: Training with Purpose and Timing

For those of you who want to challenge yourself on a deeper level, physically, mentally, and spiritually, it's time to introduce the concept of **Periodisation.**

In the world of elite sport, periodisation is a method of structuring training into phases or "blocks." Each block has a specific goal: build muscle, improve endurance, burn fat, increase power, or recover and reset. It's designed to bring out your peak performance at the right time, and it works because the body, like the mind, thrives on cycles of challenge, adaptation, and recovery.

Now here's where it gets powerful for you.

You don't have to be a professional athlete to use periodisation in your life. In fact, I believe it's one of the smartest ways to bring discipline, structure, and awareness into your routine, because it trains both your body and your mind to work in harmony.

How to Apply It:

- **Phase 1: Build the Foundation.**

Focus on strength, mobility, and nutrition. This is where you give your body what it needs to rebuild and fortify itself. It's about laying bricks, not chasing aesthetics.

Sleep well. Eat clean. Move often.

- **Phase 2: Condition and Shape.**

Once your foundation's set, gradually increase the intensity. Incorporate cardio, circuits, interval training. Focus on discipline. This isn't about killing yourself — it's about consistency under pressure.

- **Phase 3: Lean and Reset.**

This is your cutting phase. Clean up your diet further, sharpen your routines, and aim for efficiency in both movement and mind. Mental clarity improves when inflammation and sluggishness drop.

- **Phase 4: Recovery and Reflection.**

No growth comes without rest. This isn't laziness, it's strategy. Your mind and body need the space to integrate your gains. Use this time for mindfulness, journaling, or light activities like walking and stretching. Reset the nervous system.

Why This Matters:

Life itself comes in seasons.

Work pressure rises and falls. Personal challenges come and go. You'll have windows where you can push harder, and times where you need to pull back. **Periodisation teaches you to work with life's rhythm, not against it.**

When you're operating from the mindful version of yourself, you'll start to recognise these windows of opportunity. You'll sense when it's time to build, when to lean out, and when to rest. And when those moments come, take them. Because those intentional leaps forward, backed by discipline and self-awareness, often become the defining turning points of your life.

Discipline isn't punishment. It's preparation. And structure isn't limitation. It's freedom.

When you learn to periodise both your physical and mental training, you create a strategy for success that isn't reactive, it's designed by you, for you.

Life Periodisation Framework: Training the AI Within

Just like physical training, your life, mind and energy work best when approached in structured, intentional phases. We weren't designed to be 'on' all the time, and when we are, performance, health, and clarity drop.

This framework teaches you to identify and honour life's seasons, to strategically use growth periods, challenge phases, and recovery windows to your advantage.

The 4 Phases of Life Periodisation

Build Phase (Prepare & Strengthen)

When: New job, new relationship, health kick, starting a project.

Focus:
- Build foundations in health, mindset, routine.
- Learn, plan, test ideas.
- Build resilience and structure.

Why: Without a solid base, stress and demands later will collapse you.

Challenge Phase (Push & Expand)

When: You feel strong, aligned, and opportunities appear.

Focus:

- Push beyond comfort: physically, mentally, emotionally.
- Take on hard projects, difficult conversations, risk stepping up.
- Increase discipline and embrace temporary discomfort.

Why: Growth only happens in tension, but not forever.

Consolidation Phase (Adapt & Integrate)

When: After a challenge, major event, or stressful season.

Focus:

- Let new habits settle and integrate.
- Reflect on lessons, wins, mistakes.
- Adjust strategy.

Why: Without consolidation, the lessons of growth phases fade.

Recovery Phase (Reset & Rebuild)

When: You're fatigued, uninspired, or life forces a pause.

Focus:

- Prioritise rest, nature, light movement, creative play.
- Detox emotionally, mentally, physically.
- Reconnect with purpose, loved ones, and self.

Why: True strength comes from your ability to stop, rest, and come back smarter.

How to Use It

- **Track your own life seasons** — journal which phase you're in right now.
- **Match your exercise, nutrition, socialising, and work demands to the phase.**
- **Avoid the mistake** of constant Challenge Phase living (burnout) or endless Recovery (stagnation).

Example 6-Week Periodisation Program

This is a simple structure to introduce **periodised living,** using planned phases of effort, recovery, and progression to build both body and mind. Adapt it to your fitness level, life demands, and goals.

Phase 1: Foundation Build (Weeks 1–2)

Goal: Wake up the body, clean up fuel, stabilise routine.

- **Training:**
    - 3–4 walks (20–40 mins) or light cardio sessions
    - 2–3 full-body strength/resistance sessions (bodyweight or light weights)
    - 1 flexibility/mobility session (stretching, yoga, or guided breathing)
- **Mind:**
    - Daily journaling (5–10 minutes)
    - 3 guided meditations per week (even a simple 5-minute session works)
- **Nutrition:**
    - Focus on hydration (2–3L daily)
    - Add 20–30g protein with each meal
    - Minimise processed sugar and heavy takeout meals

Why: You're laying the groundwork. Waking the system, not breaking it.

Phase 2: Build & Condition (Weeks 3–4)

Goal: Increase load, build mental and physical resilience.

- **Training:**

- 2–3 cardio sessions (intervals or longer steady pace)
- 3 resistance training sessions (add weight or reps from phase 1)
- 1–2 flexibility/mobility or recovery sessions

- **Mind:**
  - Gratitude journaling daily (3 things you're grateful for)
  - Introduce visualisation practice before workouts or bed (3–5 mins)

- **Nutrition:**
  - Increase protein intake to support muscle repair
  - Introduce fruit/veg with every meal
  - Clean, energy-rich breakfasts (fruit first to wake up the system, then protein)

Why: Build physical capacity while training discipline and consistency.

Phase 3: Lean & Reset (Weeks 5–6)

Goal: Sharpen routines, dial in recovery, notice patterns.

- **Training:**
  - 3 strength or resistance sessions (higher reps, lighter load)

- 3–4 cardio sessions (longer walks, intervals, cycling, swimming)
- 1–2 mindfulness-focused activities (yoga, nature walks, breathing work)

- **Mind:**
  - Reflect on what's improved — energy, clarity, discipline
  - Journal setbacks and how you bounced back

- **Nutrition:**
  - Cleanest eating phase, mostly whole foods
  - Prioritise sleep (7–8 hours)
  - Reduce alcohol and sugar where possible

Why: Clean out inflammation. Create mental clarity. Reset for your next cycle.

Key Notes:

- If life gets hectic — swap a cardio for a walk.
- If motivation drops — reflect, reset, don't quit.
- This isn't punishment; it's building a new operating system.

Weight Training Structure, and Nutrition

A Thought Before We Begin Training and Nutrition

Before we dive into the training and nutrition section, I want to make something clear — this is not here to tell you what you *should* be doing. Most of you already have routines, habits, and preferences when it comes to food, exercise, and recovery. And if what you're doing is working, keep going. What you'll find here is simply a guide, a place to start if you're looking to make a shift, refine your process, or reignite motivation. Sometimes we just need a new reference point to trigger change. Use this as fuel to think differently, experiment with adjustments, and see how small tweaks can compound into powerful, lasting improvements.

Why the below superset?

Pairing exercises for opposing muscle groups (legs to upper body and back again) improves circulation, increases oxygen delivery to working muscles, enhances calorie burn, and sharpens your AI's adaptability to shifting demands.

It also keeps your workouts efficient and engaging.

Day 1 — Full Body Focus

5 Sets Superset

- **Leg Press / Squats**

Primary movers: quads, glutes, hamstrings, core stabilisers.

- Lat Pulldown / Pull-ups

Back, biceps, grip strength, and posture correction.

- Upright Rows

Shoulders, traps, and upper back posture.

- Abs, Obliques (Side Planks / Russian Twists /

5 Sets Superset

- Deadlifts / Walking Lunges

Posterior chain, legs, glutes, grip, and full body stability.

- Bench Press / Push-ups

Chest, shoulders, triceps.

- Abs Forward Motion (Leg Raises / Crunches / Hanging Knee Tucks)

Day 2 — Power & Athletic Movement

5 Sets Superset

- Step-ups / Box Jumps / Bulgarian Split Squats
- Seated Row / Bent Over Dumbbell Raises
- Dumbbell Flys / Incline Chest Press
- Abs Variation (Planks / Bicycle Crunches) 5 Sets Superset

- **Hamstring Curls / Romanian Deadlifts**
- **Overhead Rows (Barbell or Cables)**
- **Biceps Curls & Triceps Dips**
- **Dumbbell Shoulder Press**
- **Abs Variation (V-Ups / Weighted Sit-ups)**

Cardio Options

Choose what suits your mood, body and available time:

- 20–30 min fast walk or incline treadmill.
- 10 min warm-up row, 10 min boxing bag rounds.
- HIIT: 30 sec sprint / 1 min walk x 6 rounds.
- Bike intervals: 1 min hard, 2 min easy x 5.

Daily Nutrition Guide

This isn't a restrictive diet, it's a **base framework** to keep your internal AI sharp, your mood stable, and your body recovering.

It's also important to build flexibility and contrast days, as life will throw you the occasional pizza, footy pie, or road trip burger, and that's all part of it.

What matters is **always returning to base**.

Pre-Breakfast

- A piece of fresh fruit (banana / apple / berries)

This wakes up the system, kicks off digestion gently.

- Black coffee or green tea.

Neuro-stimulant to wake up the brain and AI.

- Light mobility stretches or breath work.

Training: Cardio or Weights

Breakfast

- **Option 1:** Eggs (boiled / scrambled) on toast
- **Option 2:** Protein shake with banana and nuts
- **Option 3:** Porridge / Weet-bix with a drizzle of honey, cinnamon, and berries

Morning Snack

- Protein bar or boiled eggs
- A small handful of almonds, walnuts, or pistachios

Lunch

- **Chicken / Salmon / Lean Beef** with steamed rice or quinoa, and stir-fry greens

- **Quick option:** 6–8 pieces of sushi
- **Salad wrap with chicken, grilled meat / falafel / tofu**

Afternoon Snack

- Greek yoghurt with nuts or granola
- Coffee or green tea
- A piece of fruit (apple, mandarin, or berries)

Dinner

- **Lean Protein:** Chicken / fish / steak
- **Steamed, roasted or stir-fried vegetables**
- **Add rice or potato** if appetite calls for it, especially if feeling very hungry

Note

Occasional cheat meal is good for contrast, at the footy pies, burgers, pizza.

The key is to **anchor yourself to your baseline,** knowing what clean eating feels like so you can return to it effortlessly.

Bonus: Grateful Pause Before Meals

A 20-second pause before eating, to give thanks for the food, the farmer who grew it, the energy it provides, **rewires your AI to register**

nourishment consciously.

This improves digestion, regulates blood sugar response, and strengthens your emotional state with every meal.

You'll eat slower, enjoy more, and train your subconscious to see food as fuel, not just comfort.

www.ingramcontent.com/pod-product-compliance
Lightning Source LLC
Chambersburg PA
CBHW071904070526
44583CB00016B/1834